This Essential Oils Journal Belongs To:

_____

A Quick Reminder

ESSENTIAL OILS ARE A LOT OF FUN WHEN USED SAFELY.

WHEN CHOOSING TO USE ESSENTIAL OILS, DO SO WITH CAUTION. ESSENTIAL OILS ARE VERY POTENT. NOT ALL OILS ARE SAFE FOR PETS, CHILDREN, THE ELDERLY, OR PREGNANT WOMEN. DOSAGE CAN VARY DEPENDING ON YOUR INDIVIDUAL HEALTH HISTORY AND NEEDS. **ALWAYS CONSULT A DOCTOR FOR APPROVAL PRIOR TO USING ESSENTIAL OILS.**

FOR DIFFUSER BLENDS: THERE ARE MANY TYPES OF PERSONAL DIFFUSERS. SOME ADD WATER AND SOME DO NOT. FOLLOW THE INSTRUCTIONS FOR YOUR DIFFUSER WHEN TESTING OUT ALL DIFFUSER BLENDS IN THIS BOOK. ALWAYS DIFFUSE IN AN OPEN AREA AND FOR NO LONGER THAN 30 MINUTES AT ONE TIME.

FOR PERFUMES: WHEN APPLYING TOPICALLY, ALWAYS DILUTE ESSENTIAL OILS. A COMMON SUGGESTED DILUTION RATIO FOR AN AVERAGE ADULT IS 1-2 DROPS OF ESSENTIAL OIL PER 1 TSP. CARRIER OIL. EXAMPLES OF CARRIER OILS INCLUDE ALMOND, AVOCADO, APRICOT KERNAL, ARGAN, GRAPESEED, JOJOBA, ROSEHIP, OR COCONUT OIL. RECIPE BLENDS IN THIS BOOK ARE BETWEEN 1%-2% DILUTION OR NO MORE THAN 12 DROPS ESSENTIAL OIL PER 1 OZ. CARRIER OIL. IT IS NOT RECOMMENDED TO EXCEED THIS RATIO.

THIS WORKBOOK IS INTENDED FOR ADULTS ONLY. USING ESSENTIAL OILS IS DONE AT YOUR OWN RISK. IF EXPERIENCING IRRITATION WHEN USING OILS, STOP USE IMMEDIATELY AND CONSULT YOUR PHYSICIAN.

BLENDS IN THIS BOOK ARE NOT INTENDED TO BE CURES FOR DISEASES. THEY SHOULD NOT BE USED IN PLACE OF STANDARD MEDICAL TREATMENT RECOMMENDED BY A LICENSCED PHYSICIAN.

Essential Oil Inventory

NAME	USED FOR	DATE OPENED	FAVORITE?

Essential Oil Inventory

NAME	USED FOR	DATE OPENED	FAVORITE?

Essential Oil Wish List

NAME	USED FOR	PRICE	KID SAFE?

My Favorite Oils

ENERGY

CALMING

SLEEP

FOCUS/CLARITY

WELLNESS

ROMANCE

ANXIETY

JOYFUL

My Oil Ratings

PURPOSE OF OIL

NAME:

MY RATING:

PURPOSE OF OIL

NAME:

MY RATING:

PURPOSE OF OIL

NAME:

MY RATING:

PURPOSE OF OIL

NAME:

MY RATING:

PURPOSE OF OIL

NAME:

MY RATING:

NOTES:

Wellness Blends

DIFFUSER BLENDS

NAME: ENERGIZING

4 DROPS PEPPERMINT

4 DROPS CINNAMON

2 DROPS ROSEMARY

NAME: EXTREME FOCUS

3 DROPS ROSEMARY

2 DROPS FRANKINCENSE

2 DROPS VETIVER

NAME: INNER CALM

3 DROPS LAVENDER

3 DROPS BERGAMOT

3 DROPS FRANKINCENSE

NAME: TRANQUILITY

3 DROPS LAVENDER

2 DROPS LIME

3 DROPS MANDARIN

NAME: CARPE DIEM

3 DROPS ROSEMARY

3 DROPS PEPPERMINT

3 DROPS FRANKINCENSE

NAME: STRESS BE GONE

3 DROPS LAVENDER

2 DROPS CHAMOMILE

2 DROPS YLANG YLANG

NAME: RELAXATION

3 DROPS BERGAMOT

3 DROPS PATCHOULI

3 DROPS YLANG YLANG

NAME: ACTIVE LIFE

2 DROPS GRAPEFRUIT

3 DROPS PEPPERMINT

3 DROPS ROSEMARY

NOTES: THERE ARE MANY TYPES OF PERSONAL DIFFUSERS.. SOME ADD WATER TO BLENDS AND SOME DO NOT. FOLLOW THE INSTRUCTIONS FOR YOUR DIFFUSER WHEN TESTING OUT ALL DIFFUSER BLENDS IN THIS BOOK. NOT ALL OILS ARE SAFE FOR PETS, CHILDREN, THE ELDERLY, OR PREGNANT WOMEN. **ALWAYS CONSULT A DOCTOR PRIOR TO USING ESSENTIAL OILS**.

Testing Out Blends

NAME:

PURPOSE:

INGREDIENTS:

DIFFUSER

INHALER

TOPICAL

OTHER

MY RATING:

NOTES:

Testing Out Blends

NAME:

PURPOSE:

INGREDIENTS:

DIFFUSER

INHALER

TOPICAL

OTHER

MY RATING:

NOTES:

My Favorite Blends

NAME:

USED FOR:

INGREDIENTS:

NOTES:

NAME:

USED FOR:

INGREDIENTS:

NOTES:

Essential Oil Recipes

NAME:

NAME:

NAME:

NAME:

NAME:

NAME:

NAME:

NAME:

My Favorite Oils

CREATIVITY

MEMORY

ATHLETIC RECOVERY

DEPRESSION RELIEF

MEDITATION

CONFIDENCE

PRODUCTIVITY

HAPPINESS

My Oil Ratings

PURPOSE OF OIL

NAME:

MY RATING:

PURPOSE OF OIL

NAME:

MY RATING:

PURPOSE OF OIL

NAME:

MY RATING:

PURPOSE OF OIL

NAME:

MY RATING:

PURPOSE OF OIL

NAME:

MY RATING:

NOTES:

Personality Blends

DIFFUSER BLENDS

NAME: CONFIDENT

2 DROPS SPEARMINT

2 DROPS TANGERINE

2 DROPS BERGAMOT

NAME: CAREFREE

5 DROPS BERGAMOT

2 DROPS PATCHOULI

2 DROPS LIME

NAME: HAPPY

2 DROPS WILD ORANGE

2 DROPS GRAPEFRUIT

2 DROPS CLOVE

NAME: INSPIRED

1 DROP ROSE

1 DROP LAVENDER

2 DROPS JUNIPER BERRY

NAME: FOCUSED

3 DROPS DOUGLAS FIR

2 DROPS LEMON

1 DROP PEPPERMINT

NAME: ENERGETIC

2 DROPS PEPPERMINT

3 DROPS GRAPEFRUIT

3 DROPS BERGAMOT

NAME: MOTIVATED

2 DROPS GRAPEFRUIT

2 DROPS CYPRESS

2 DROPS LIME

NAME: PEACEFUL

2 DROPS FRANKINCENSE

2 DROPS WHITE FIR

2 DROPS LAVENDER

NOTES:

Testing Out Blends

NAME:

INGREDIENTS:

PURPOSE:

DIFFUSER

INHALER

TOPICAL

OTHER

MY RATING:

NOTES:

Testing Out Blends

NAME: **PURPOSE**:

INGREDIENTS:

DIFFUSER

INHALER

TOPICAL

OTHER

MY RATING:

NOTES:

My Favorite Blends

NAME: USED FOR:

INGREDIENTS:

NOTES:

NAME: USED FOR:

INGREDIENTS:

NOTES:

Happiness Blends

DIFFUSER BLENDS

NAME: SIP OF SUNSHINE

3 DROPS WILD ORANGE

3 DROPS FRANKINCENSE

1 DROP CINNAMON

NAME: INNER PEACE

2 DROPS PEPPERMINT

2 DROPS LAVENDER

2 DROPS WILD ORANGE

NAME: WITH PURPOSE

3 DROPS LEMON

2 DROPS OREGANO

2 DROPS CLOVE

NAME: BOOSTER

2 DROPS LAVENDER

3 DROPS SWEET ORANGE

3 DROPS PEPPERMINT

NAME: GENTLE SOUL

3 DROPS BERGAMOT

2 DROPS GERANIUM

3 DROPS LAVENDER

NAME: ZONED OUT

2 DROPS ROSEMARY

2 DROPS CINNAMON

1 DROP CLOVE

NAME: LAUGHTER

3 DROPS LEMON

3 DROPS TANGERINE

2 DROPS TEA TREE

NAME: MINDFULNESS

3 DROPS LAVENDER

3 DROPS BERGAMOT

1 DROP CLOVE

NOTES:

Testing Out Blends

NAME:

PURPOSE:

INGREDIENTS:

DIFFUSER

INHALER

TOPICAL

OTHER

MY RATING:

NOTES:

Testing Out Blends

NAME:

PURPOSE:

INGREDIENTS:

DIFFUSER

INHALER

TOPICAL

OTHER

MY RATING:

NOTES:

My Favorite Blends

NAME:

USED FOR:

INGREDIENTS:

NOTES:

NAME:

USED FOR:

INGREDIENTS:

NOTES:

Essential Oil Recipes

NAME:

NAME:

NAME:

NAME:

NAME:

NAME:

NAME:

NAME:

Well Rested Blends

DIFFUSER BLENDS

NAME: SWEET LULLABY

3 DROPS JUNIPER BERRY

3 DROPS CHAMOMILE

3 DROPS LAVENDER

NAME: DEEP CALM

4 DROPS CEDARWOOD

3 DROPS LAVENDER

1 DROP VETIVER

NAME: SO DREAMY

2 DROPS FRANKINCENSE

3 DROPS VETIVER

2 DROPS LAVENDER

NAME: PEACEFUL SLUMBER

3 DROPS FRANKINCENSE

2 DROPS LAVENDER

2 DROPS CHAMOMILE

NAME: SWEET DREAMS

3 DROPS LAVENDER

2 DROPS MARJORAM

2 DROPS ORANGE

NAME: DREAMCATCHER

3 DROPS LEMON

3 DROPS LAVENDER

2 DROPS PEPPERMINT

NAME: THE SANDMAN

5 DROPS PEPPERMINT

4 DROPS EUCALYPTUS

2 DROPS MYRRH

NAME: WELL RESTED

3 DROPS LAVENDER

3 DROPS CHAMOMILE

1 DROP CLOVE

NOTES:

Testing Out Blends

NAME:

PURPOSE:

INGREDIENTS:

DIFFUSER

INHALER

TOPICAL

OTHER

MY RATING:

NOTES:

My Favorite Blends

NAME: USED FOR:

INGREDIENTS:

NOTES:

NAME: USED FOR:

INGREDIENTS:

NOTES:

Essential Oil Recipes

NAME:

NAME:

NAME:

NAME:

NAME:

NAME:

NAME:

NAME:

My Favorite Oils

NASAL CONGESTION

SORE MUSCLES

HEADACHE

CHEST CONGESTION

SKIN CONDITIONS

INDIGESTION

FEVER/CHILLS

NAUSEA

My Oil Ratings

PURPOSE OF OIL

NAME:

MY RATING:

PURPOSE OF OIL

NAME:

MY RATING:

PURPOSE OF OIL

NAME:

MY RATING:

PURPOSE OF OIL

NAME:

MY RATING:

PURPOSE OF OIL

NAME:

MY RATING:

NOTES:

Lavender Blends

DIFFUSER BLENDS

NAME: SEA BREEZE

2 DROPS LAVENDER

3 DROPS LIME

1 DROP SPEARMINT

NAME: OCEAN BREEZE:

4 DROPS LAVENDER

3 DROPS ROSEMARY

2 DROPS LEMONGRASS

NAME: COOL DOWN

4 DROPS SPEARMINT

2 DROPS LAVENDER

2 DROPS PEPPERMINT

NAME: LAVENDER MINT

4 DROPS LAVENDER

3 DROPS PEPPERMINT

1 DROP VETIVER

NAME: PEACEFUL MOMENT

3 DROPS LAVENDER

3 DROPS VETIVER

2 DROPS YLANG-YLANG

NAME: CLEAN AIR

3 DROPS LAVENDER

3 DROPS TANGERINE

3 DROPS EUCALYPTUS

NAME: CREATIVE SPARK

3 DROPS LAVENDER

3 DROPS SWEET ORANGE

1 DROP PEPPERMINT

NAME: STUDY SESSION

2 DROPS LAVENDER

3 DROPS BERGAMOT

2 DROPS ROSEMARY

NOTES:

Testing Out Blends

NAME: **PURPOSE**:

INGREDIENTS:

DIFFUSER

INHALER

TOPICAL

OTHER

MY RATING:

NOTES:

Testing Out Blends

NAME:

PURPOSE:

INGREDIENTS:

DIFFUSER

INHALER

TOPICAL

OTHER

MY RATING:

NOTES:

My Favorite Blends

NAME:

USED FOR:

INGREDIENTS:

NOTES:

NAME:

USED FOR:

INGREDIENTS:

NOTES:

Essential Oil Recipes

NAME:

NAME:

NAME:

NAME:

NAME:

NAME:

NAME:

NAME:

My Favorite Oils

BATHROOM

POTPOURRI

LAUNDRY

KITCHEN

FLOORS

BUG DETERRENT

HAIR

BEAUTY

My Oil Ratings

PURPOSE OF OIL

NAME:

MY RATING:

PURPOSE OF OIL

NAME:

MY RATING:

PURPOSE OF OIL

NAME:

MY RATING:

PURPOSE OF OIL

NAME:

MY RATING:

PURPOSE OF OIL

NAME:

MY RATING:

NOTES:

Clean House Blends

DIFFUSER BLENDS

NAME: SPARKLY CLEAN

3 DROPS LEMON

3 DROPS PEPPERMINT

3 DROPS EUCALYPTUS

NAME: NICE & TIDY

3 DROPS EUCALYPTUS

3 DROPS WILD ORANGE

3 DROPS LIME

NAME: FRESH SCENT

3 DROPS LEMON

3 DROPS EUCALYPTUS

3 DROPS LIME

NAME: ELEGANT HOME

1 DROP ROSE

1 DROP CARDAMOM

2 DROPS WILD ORANGE

NAME: DECLUTTERING

4 DROPS LEMON

3 DROPS LEMONGRASS

2 DROPS PEPPERMINT

NAME: SPRING CLEANING

4 DROPS LEMON

3 DROPS LAVENDER

2 DROPS ROSEMARY

NAME: GLOSSY FINISH

4 DROPS FRANKINCENSE

4 DROPS CYPRESS

2 DROPS YLANG-YLANG

NAME: THE HOUSEKEEPER

2 DROPS CINNAMON

2 DROPS CARDAMOM

2 DROPS LEMOM

NOTES:

Testing Out Blends

NAME: _____

PURPOSE:

INGREDIENTS:

DIFFUSER

INHALER

TOPICAL

OTHER

MY RATING:

NOTES:

Testing Out Blends

NAME: **PURPOSE:**

INGREDIENTS:

DIFFUSER

INHALER

TOPICAL

OTHER

MY RATING:

NOTES:

My Favorite Blends

NAME:

USED FOR:

INGREDIENTS:

NOTES:

NAME:

USED FOR:

INGREDIENTS:

NOTES:

Essential Oil Recipes

NAME:

NAME:

NAME:

NAME:

NAME:

NAME:

NAME:

NAME:

Day to Day Blends

DIFFUSER BLENDS

NAME: SLEEP TIME

4 DROPS LAVENDER

4 DROPS CEDARWOOD

3 DROPS CHAMOMILE

NAME: ANTI-STRESS

4 DROPS BERGAMOT

4 DROPS FRANKINCENSE

1 DROP PEPPERMINT

NAME: ALLERGY FIGHTER

3 DROPS LAVENDER

3 DROPS LEMON

3 DROPS PEPPERMINT

NAME: CONCENTRATION

4 DROPS LAVENDER

4 DROPS TEA TREE OIL

4 DROPS FRANKINCENSE

NAME: COMBAT NAUSEA

3 DROPS GINGER

5 DROPS PEPPERMINT

1 DROP FRANKINCENSE

NAME: HEADACHES

2 DROPS FRANKINCENSE

2 DROPS LAVENDER

4 DROPS PEPPERMINT

NAME: BREATHE EASY

4 DROPS PEPPERMINT

2 DROPS EUCALYPTUS

2 DROPS LEMON

NAME: IMMUNE BOOST

2 DROPS FRANKINCENSE

5 DROPS LEMON

2 DROPS PEPPERMINT

NOTES:

My Favorite Oils

VALENTINE'S DAY

SPRING

SUMMER

AUTUMN

HALLOWEEN

WINTER

CHRISTMAS

NEW YEAR'S

My Oil Ratings

PURPOSE OF OIL

NAME:

MY RATING:

PURPOSE OF OIL

NAME:

MY RATING:

PURPOSE OF OIL

NAME:

MY RATING:

PURPOSE OF OIL

NAME:

MY RATING:

PURPOSE OF OIL

NAME:

MY RATING:

NOTES:

Spring Blends

DIFFUSER BLENDS

NAME: WELCOME SPRING

2 DROPS GERANIUM

2 DROPS LEMON

2 DROPS GRAPEFRUIT

NAME: SPRING GARDEN

2 DROPS BASIL

2 DROPS PEPPERMINT

2 DROPS LIME

NAME: FRESH & CLEAN

4 DROPS GRAPEFRUIT

3 DROPS PEPPERMINT

3 DROPS CLARY SAGE

NAME: FLOWER BASKET

5 DROPS CLARY SAGE

3 DROPS LAVENDER

2 DROPS GERANIUM

NAME: SPRING PETALS

2 DROPS YLANG YLANG

2 DROPS PEPPERMINT

2 DROPS LEMON

NAME: MOTHER NATURE

3 DROPS PEPPERMINT

3 DROPS LAVENDER

3 DROPS LEMON

NAME: RENEWAL

2 DROPS LAVENDER

3 DROPS LEMON

3 DROPS ROSEMARY

NAME: GOOD MORNING

3 DROPS CINNAMON

2 DROPS TANGERINE

1 DROP LEMON

NOTES:

Testing Out Blends

NAME: **PURPOSE**:

INGREDIENTS: DIFFUSER

                                         INHALER

                                         TOPICAL

                                         OTHER

                                MY RATING:

NOTES:

Testing Out Blends

NAME: **PURPOSE:**

INGREDIENTS:

DIFFUSER

INHALER

TOPICAL

OTHER

MY RATING:

NOTES:

My Favorite Blends

NAME:

USED FOR:

INGREDIENTS:

NOTES:

NAME:

USED FOR:

INGREDIENTS:

NOTES:

Summer Blends

DIFFUSER BLENDS

NAME: SWEET SUNSHINE

- 3 DROPS LEMONGRASS
- 2 DROPS ORANGE
- 1 DROP PEPPERMINT

NAME: SUNNY DAYS

- 3 DROPS TANGERINE
- 3 DROPS LEMON
- 1 DROP PEPPERMINT

NAME: HAMMOCK TIME

- 2 DROPS LAVENDER
- 2 DROPS CEDARWOOD
- 2 DROPS WILD ORANGE

NAME: CITRUS TWIST

- 2 DROPS TANGERINE
- 2 DROPS GRAPEFRUIT
- 2 DROPS LEMON

NAME: SUMMER LOVING

- 2 DROPS JUNIPER BERRY
- 2 DROPS GRAPEFRUIT
- 2 DROPS WILD ORANGE

NAME: BEACH TOWN

- 3 DROPS BERGAMOT
- 3 DROPS LAVENDER
- 3 DROPS ROSEMARY

NAME: BEACH MEMORIES

- 2 DROPS SPEARMINT
- 3 DROPS TANGERINE
- 2 DROPS BERGAMOT

NAME: SUN-KISSED

- 2 DROPS TEA TREE
- 2 DROPS LEMON
- 2 DROPS LIME

NOTES:

Testing Out Blends

NAME:

PURPOSE:

INGREDIENTS:

DIFFUSER

INHALER

TOPICAL

OTHER

MY RATING:

NOTES:

Testing Out Blends

NAME: **PURPOSE:**

INGREDIENTS:

	PURPOSE
	DIFFUSER
	INHALER
	TOPICAL
	OTHER

MY RATING:

NOTES:

My Favorite Blends

NAME: USED FOR:

INGREDIENTS:

NOTES:

NAME: USED FOR:

INGREDIENTS:

NOTES:

Autumn Blends

DIFFUSER BLENDS

NAME: PUMPKIN SPICE

5 DROPS CINNAMON

2 DROPS NUTMEG

3 DROPS CLOVE

NAME: SNICKERDOODLE

5 DROPS STRESS AWAY

3 DROPS CINNAMON

2 DROPS NUTMEG

NAME: FLANNEL SHEETS

5 DROPS BLACK SPRUCE

4 DROPS STRESS AWAY

4 DROPS ORANGE

NAME: HAND-KNIT SWEATER

5 DROPS ORANGE

4 DROPS THIEVES

1 DROP GINGER

NAME: WARM CIDER

4 DROPS ORANGE

3 DROPS CINNAMON

3 DROPS GINGER

NAME: CHANGING LEAVES

5 DROPS CLOVE

5 DROPS CEDARWOOD

5 DROPS ORANGE

NAME: GIVING THANKS

5 DROPS CINNAMON

3 DROPS ORANGE

2 DROPS NUTMEG

NAME: AUTUMN BREEZE

4 DROPS ORANGE

2 DROPS CLOVE

1 DROP LEMON

NOTES:

Testing Out Blends

NAME:

PURPOSE:

INGREDIENTS:

DIFFUSER

INHALER

TOPICAL

OTHER

MY RATING:

NOTES:

Testing Out Blends

NAME:

PURPOSE:

INGREDIENTS:

DIFFUSER

INHALER

TOPICAL

OTHER

MY RATING:

NOTES:

My Favorite Blends

NAME: USED FOR:

INGREDIENTS:

NOTES:

NAME: USED FOR:

INGREDIENTS:

NOTES:

Winter Blends

DIFFUSER BLENDS

NAME: WINTER CITRUS

2 DROPS PEPPERMINT

2 DROPS LEMONGRASS

2 DROPS TANGERINE

NAME: SNOW DAYS

2 DROPS CEDARWOOD

2 DROPS THIEVES

2 DROPS CITRUS

NAME: CLASSIC WINTER

2 DROPS CEDARWOOD

2 DROPS LAVENDER

2 DROPS ROSEMARY

NAME: COZY HOME

2 DROPS BERGAMOT

2 DROPS ORANGE

2 DROPS THIEVES

NAME: SNOWFLAKE

2 DROPS LAVENDER

2 DROPS LEMON

2 DROPS PEPPERMINT

NAME: WINTER SOLSTICE

5 DROPS PINE

4 DROPS PEPPERMINT

2 DROPS CINNAMON

NAME: HOLIDAY BAKING

2 DROPS CASSIA

2 DROPS VETIVER

2 DROPS LAVENDER

NAME: WINTER MEMORIES

2 DROPS BERGAMOT

2 DROPS WILD ORANGE

2 DROPS EUCALYPTUS

NOTES:

Testing Out Blends

NAME:

PURPOSE:

INGREDIENTS:

DIFFUSER

INHALER

TOPICAL

OTHER

MY RATING:

NOTES:

Testing Out Blends

NAME:

PURPOSE:

INGREDIENTS:

DIFFUSER

INHALER

TOPICAL

OTHER

MY RATING:

NOTES:

My Favorite Blends

NAME: USED FOR:

INGREDIENTS:

NOTES:

NAME: USED FOR:

INGREDIENTS:

NOTES:

Holiday Blends

DIFFUSER BLENDS

NAME: DECK THE HALLS

4 DROPS PINE

2 DROPS BLUE SPRUCE

2 DROPS CEDARWOOD

NAME: CANDY CANE

4 DROPS PEPPERMINT

3 DROPS BERGAMOT

1 DROP WILD ORANGE

NAME: SUGAR PLUM FAIRY

3 DROPS WILD ORANGE

2 DROPS DOUGLAS FIR

2 DROPS PEPPERMINT

NAME: YULETIDE BLESSING

5 DROPS THIEVES

2 DROPS FRANKINCENSE

2 DROPS WILD ORANGE

NAME: SNOW ANGELS

4 DROPS CEDARWOOD

3 FRESH CITRUS

1 DROP FRANKINCENSE

NAME: SPICED CIDER

3 DROPS WILD ORANGE

2 DROPS CINNAMON BARK

1 DROP CLOVE

NAME: MERRY & BRIGHT

3 DROPS LEMON

2 DROPS DOUGLAS FIR

2 DROPS CINNAMON

NAME: GINGERBREAD MAN

4 DROPS GINGER

2 DROPS CLOVES

2 DROPS CINNAMON

NOTES:

Essential Oil Recipes

NAME:

NAME:

NAME:

NAME:

NAME:

NAME:

NAME:

NAME:

Perfume Blend Suggestions

ROLL-ON BLENDS TO BE DILUTED WITH 1 OZ. CARRIER OIL

NAME: SUMMER NIGHTS

3 DROPS WILD ORANGE

4 DROPS GERANIUM

2 DROPS SANDALWOOD

NAME: EXOTIC ORCHARD

3 DROPS GRAPEFRUIT

4 DROPS JUNIPER BERRY

1 DROP MYRRH

NAME: FREE LOVE

5 DROPS BERGAMOT

3 DROPS CLARY SAGE

3 DROPS PATCHOULI

NAME: TROPICAL RADIANCE

3 DROPS SWEET ORANGE

4 DROPS NEROLI

3 DROPS CEDARWOOD

NAME: TABLE FOR TWO

5 DROPS LAVENDER

4 DROPS SWEET ORANGE

1 DROP YLANG-YLANG

NAME: TWILIGHT GARDEN

4 DROPS BERGAMOT

4 DROPS GERANIUM

2 DROPS VETIVER

NAME: 5 O'CLOCK SHADOW

6 DROPS BERGAMOT

4 DROPS WHITE FIR

1 DROP CLOVE

NAME: GREAT OUTDOORS

3 DROPS EUCALYPTUS

5 DROPS CYPRESS

4 DROPS VETIVER

NOTES: EXAMPLES OF CARRIER OILS ARE ALMOND,, APRICOT KERNEL, GRAPESEED, ROSEHIP,, OR COCONUT OIL. TYPICAL DILUTION IS 1-2 DROPS ESSENTIAL OIL FOR 1 TSP CARRIER OIL. DILUTION INSTRUCTIONS ARE FOR THE AVERAGE PERSON AND NOT FOR PREGNANT WOMEN, CHILDREN, PETS, OR THE ELDERLY. **ALWAYS CONSULT A DOCTOR PRIOR TO USING ESSENTIAL OILS.** IF IRRITATION OCCURS, DISCONTINUE USE.

Testing Out Blends

NAME:

PURPOSE:

INGREDIENTS:

DIFFUSER

INHALER

TOPICAL

OTHER

MY RATING:

NOTES:

Testing Out Blends

NAME: **PURPOSE:**

INGREDIENTS:

DIFFUSER

INHALER

TOPICAL

OTHER

MY RATING:

NOTES:

My Favorite Perfume Blends

PERFUME BLENDS

NAME:

NAME:

NAME:

NAME:

NAME:

NAME:

NAME:

NAME:

NOTES:

My Favorite Magical Oils

THE GODS

THE GODDESSES

LUCK

MONEY

LOVE

INSPIRATION

DIVINATION

PROTECTION

My Favorite Magical Oils

WELLNESS

COURAGE

DEVOTION

JUSTICE

EARTH

AIR

WATER

FIRE

Magical Blends

DIFFUSER BLENDS

NAME: IMBOLC EVENING

3 DROPS CEDARWOOD

3 DROPS LAVENDER

1 DROP NEROLI

NAME: BELTANE BLISS

4 DROPS GERANIUM

4 DROPS JASMINE

4 DROPS FRANKINCENSE

NAME: THE FIRST HARVEST

3 DROPS SANDALWOOD

2 DROPS FRANKINCENSE

2 DROPS ROSE

NAME: SAMHAIN BLESSINGS

4 DROPS CINNAMON

3 DROPS GINGER

2 DROPS SAGE

NAME: SPRING FEVER

4 DROPS JASMINE

2 DROPS ROSE

2 DROPS PATCHOULI

NAME: MIDSUMMER MAGIC

5 DROPS LAVENDER

3 DROPS SWEET ORANGE

2 DROPS GERANIUM

NAME: AUTUMN ARRIVAL

3 DROPS ORANGE

2 DROPS PINE

2 DROPS CINNAMON

NAME: YULE FIRE

4 DROPS PINE

2 DROPS CINNAMON

1 DROP NUTMEG

NOTES:

Testing Out Blends

NAME:

PURPOSE:

INGREDIENTS:

DIFFUSER

INHALER

TOPICAL

OTHER

MY RATING:

NOTES:

Testing Out Blends

NAME:

PURPOSE:

INGREDIENTS:

DIFFUSER

INHALER

TOPICAL

OTHER

MY RATING:

NOTES:

Magical Essential Oil Recipes

NAME:

NAME:

NAME:

NAME:

NAME:

NAME:

NAME:

NAME:

My Journey With Essential Oils

How have I grown?

Essential Oil Inventory

NAME	USED FOR	DATE OPENED	FAVORITE?

Essential Oil Inventory

NAME	USED FOR	DATE OPENED	FAVORITE?

Essential Oil Wish List

NAME	USED FOR	PRICE	KID SAFE?

My Favorite Oils

ENERGY

CALMING

SLEEP

FOCUS/CLARITY

WELLNESS

ROMANCE

ANXIETY

JOY

My Oil Ratings

PURPOSE OF OIL

NAME:

MY RATING:

PURPOSE OF OIL

NAME:

MY RATING:

PURPOSE OF OIL

NAME:

MY RATING:

PURPOSE OF OIL

NAME:

MY RATING:

PURPOSE OF OIL

NAME:

MY RATING:

NOTES:

Wellness Blends

DIFFUSER BLENDS

NAME: EARLY BIRD

3 DROPS BERGAMOT

2 DROPS PEPPERMINT

1 DROP GRAPFRUIT

NAME: PRODIGY

4 DROPS ROSEMARY

3 DROPS BASIL

5 DROPS CYPRESS

NAME: ZEN

3 DROPS LAVENDER

3 DROPS BERGAMOT

3 DROPS GERANIUM

NAME: AT EASE

3 DROPS LAVENDER

2 DROPS YLANG-YLANG

3 DROPS PATCHOULI

NAME: LOVER OF LIFE

3 DROPS ORANGE

3 DROPS LIME

3 DROPS FRANKINCENSE

NAME: FREE SPIRIT

3 DROPS BERGAMOT

2 DROPS PATCHOULI

2 DROPS YLANG YLANG

NAME: SERENITY

3 DROPS LAVENDER

3 DROPS ORANGE

3 DROPS YLANG YLANG

NAME: READY FOR ACTION

2 DROPS PEPPERMINT

3 DROPS ORANGE

3 DROPS FRANKINCENSE

NOTES:

Testing Out Blends

NAME:

PURPOSE:

INGREDIENTS:

DIFFUSER

INHALER

TOPICAL

OTHER

MY RATING:

NOTES:

Testing Out Blends

NAME: **PURPOSE:**

INGREDIENTS:

DIFFUSER

INHALER

TOPICAL

OTHER

MY RATING:

NOTES:

My Favorite Blends

NAME:

USED FOR:

INGREDIENTS:

NOTES:

NAME:

USED FOR:

INGREDIENTS:

NOTES:

Essential Oil Recipes

NAME:

NAME:

NAME:

NAME:

NAME:

NAME:

NAME:

NAME:

My Favorite Oils

CREATIVITY

MEMORY

ATHLETIC RECOVERY

DEPRESSION RELIEF

MEDITATION

CONFIDENCE

PRODUCTIVITY

HAPPINESS

My Oil Ratings

PURPOSE OF OIL

NAME:

MY RATING:

PURPOSE OF OIL

NAME:

MY RATING:

PURPOSE OF OIL

NAME:

MY RATING:

PURPOSE OF OIL

NAME:

MY RATING:

PURPOSE OF OIL

NAME:

MY RATING:

NOTES:

Personality Blends

DIFFUSER BLENDS

NAME: CONFIDENT STRIDE

2 DROPS FRANKINCENSE

2 DROPS SWEET ORANGE

2 DROPS ROSEMARY

NAME: LASER BEAM

2 DROPS LAVENDER

1 DROP BLACK PEPPER

1 DROP SANDLEWOOD

NAME: NO CARES

3 DROPS ORANGE

2 DROPS LAVENDER

1 DROP YLANG-YLANG

NAME: UPBEAT

3 DROPS PEPPERMINT

3 DROPS GRAPEFRUIT

3 DROPS BERGAMOT

NAME: INNER JOY

2 DROPS WILD ORANGE

2 DROPS FRANKINCENSE

2 DROPS BERGAMOT

NAME: TENACIOUS

6 DROPS LEMON

4 DROPS BASIL

3 DROPS ROSEMARY

NAME: DIVINELY INSPIRED

1 DROP SANDLEWOOD

1 DROP CEDARWOOD

2 DROPS FRANKINCENSE

NAME: CLOUD 9

5 DROPS CLARY-SAGE

3 DROPS GERANIUM

3 DROPS VETIVER

NOTES:

Testing Out Blends

NAME: **PURPOSE:**

INGREDIENTS:

DIFFUSER

INHALER

TOPICAL

OTHER

MY RATING:

NOTES:

Testing Out Blends

NAME:

PURPOSE:

INGREDIENTS:

DIFFUSER

INHALER

TOPICAL

OTHER

MY RATING:

NOTES:

My Favorite Blends

NAME:

USED FOR:

INGREDIENTS:

NOTES:

NAME:

USED FOR:

INGREDIENTS:

NOTES:

Happiness Blends

DIFFUSER BLENDS

NAME: CHEERFUL TUNE

5 DROPS WILD ORANGE

3 DROPS ROSEMARY

3 DROPS LEMON

NAME: CALM & CENTERED

4 DROPS MANDARIN

3 DROPS LIME

2 DROPS LAVENDER

NAME: DETERMINED

4 DROPS ORANGE

3 DROPS CINNAMON

2 DROPS ROSEMARY

NAME: PICK-ME-UP

2 DROPS LAVENDER

3 DROPS SWEET ORANGE

3 DROPS PEPPERMINT

NAME: STRAIGHT ARROW

3 DROPS LAVENDER

2 DROPS BERGAMOT

1 DROPS VANILLA

NAME: EASY-GOING

5 DROPS BERGAMOT

3 DROPS LAVENDER

3 DROPS PATCHOULI

NAME: BELLY LAUGHS

4 DROPS GRAPEFRUIT

2 DROPS LEMON

2 DROPS LAVENDER

NAME: GET GROUNDED

4 DROPS LAVENDER

2 DROPS BERGAMOT

2 DROPS ROSEMARY

NOTES:

Testing Out Blends

NAME:

PURPOSE:

INGREDIENTS:

DIFFUSER

INHALER

TOPICAL

OTHER

MY RATING:

NOTES:

Testing Out Blends

NAME:

PURPOSE:

INGREDIENTS:

DIFFUSER

INHALER

TOPICAL

OTHER

MY RATING:

NOTES:

My Favorite Blends

NAME:

USED FOR:

INGREDIENTS:

NOTES:

NAME:

USED FOR:

INGREDIENTS:

NOTES:

Essential Oil Recipes

NAME:

NAME:

NAME:

NAME:

NAME:

NAME:

NAME:

NAME:

Well Rested Blends

DIFFUSER BLENDS

NAME: SWEET SEDATIVE

3 DROPS SWEET ORANGE

3 DROPS YLANG-YLANG

3 DROPS LAVENDER

NAME: HEAVY SLEEPER

1 DROPS VALERIAN

3 DROPS VETIVER

2 DROPS LAVENDER

NAME: COUNT NO SHEEP

3 DROPS LAVENDER

2 DROPS CLARY-SAGE

2 DROPS VETIVER

NAME: SLUMBER PARTY

5 DROPS LAVENDER

3 DROPS CLARY-SAGE

2 DROPS VALERIAN

NAME: DREAM WORLD

3 DROPS CLARY-SAGE

3 DROPS YLANG-YLANG

3 DROPS FRANKINCENSE

NAME: ENCHANTED NIGHT

4 DROPS LAVENDER

3 DROPS YLANG-YLANG

2 DROPS JASMINE

NAME: MIDNIGHT MELODY

5 DROPS CEDARWOOD

3 DROPS VETIVER

2 DROPS SWEET ORANGE

NAME: BEDTIME STORY

4 DROPS EUCALYPTUS

3 DROPS LAVENDER

3 DROP ORANGE

NOTES:

Testing Out Blends

NAME: _____

PURPOSE: _____

INGREDIENTS:

DIFFUSER

INHALER

TOPICAL

OTHER

MY RATING:

NOTES:

Testing Out Blends

NAME:

PURPOSE:

INGREDIENTS:

DIFFUSER

INHALER

TOPICAL

OTHER

MY RATING:

NOTES:

My Favorite Blends

NAME: USED FOR:

INGREDIENTS:

NOTES:

NAME: USED FOR:

INGREDIENTS:

NOTES:

Essential Oil Recipes

NAME:

NAME:

NAME:

NAME:

NAME:

NAME:

NAME:

NAME:

My Favorite Oils

NASAL CONGESTION

SORE MUSCLES

HEADACHE

CHEST CONGESTION

SKIN CONDITIONS

INDIGESTION

FEVER/CHILLS

NAUSEA

My Oil Ratings

PURPOSE OF OIL

NAME:

MY RATING:

PURPOSE OF OIL

NAME:

MY RATING:

PURPOSE OF OIL

NAME:

MY RATING:

PURPOSE OF OIL

NAME:

MY RATING:

PURPOSE OF OIL

NAME:

MY RATING:

NOTES:

Peppermint Blends

DIFFUSER BLENDS

NAME: JINGLE BELLS

4 DROPS PEPPERMINT

3 DROPS ORANGE

3 DROPS CINNAMON

NAME: DEEP RELIEF

2 DROPS PEPPERMINT

2 DROPS LAVENDER

2 DROPS LEMON

NAME: TRUE COMFORT

3 DROPS PEPPERMINT

3 DROPS EUCALYPTUS

3 DROPS SWEET ORANGE

NAME: MOUNTAIN MELODY

4 DROPS PEPPERMINT

2 DROPS BERGAMOT

1 DROP CINNAMON

NAME: FRESH START

4 DROPS PEPPERMINT

3 DROPS LEMON

2 DROPS FRANKINCENSE

NAME: SUPERHERO

2 DROPS PEPPERMINT

2 DROPS FRANKINCENSE

2 DROPS WILD ORANGE

NAME: SMOOTH MOVE

4 DROPS PEPPERMINT

3 DROPS LEMON

2 DROPS ROSEMARY

NAME: COAT OF ARMOR

2 DROPS PEPPERMINT

3 DROPS ORANGE

4 DROPS FRANKINCENSE

NOTES:

Testing Out Blends

NAME:

PURPOSE:

INGREDIENTS:

DIFFUSER

INHALER

TOPICAL

OTHER

MY RATING:

NOTES:

Testing Out Blends

NAME:

PURPOSE:

INGREDIENTS:

DIFFUSER

INHALER

TOPICAL

OTHER

MY RATING:

NOTES:

My Favorite Blends

NAME:

USED FOR:

INGREDIENTS:

NOTES:

NAME:

USED FOR:

INGREDIENTS:

NOTES:

Essential Oil Recipes

NAME:

NAME:

NAME:

NAME:

NAME:

NAME:

NAME:

NAME:

My Favorite Oils

BATHROOM

POTPOURRI

LAUNDRY

KITCHEN

FLOORS

BUG DETERRENT

HAIR

BEAUTY

My Oil Ratings

PURPOSE OF OIL

NAME:

MY RATING:

PURPOSE OF OIL

NAME:

MY RATING:

PURPOSE OF OIL

NAME:

MY RATING:

PURPOSE OF OIL

NAME:

MY RATING:

PURPOSE OF OIL

NAME:

MY RATING:

NOTES:

Clean House Blends

DIFFUSER BLENDS

NAME: SPRING CLEAN

5 DROPS JASMINE

3 DROPS ROSE

2 DROPS LAVENDER

NAME: SO FRESH

4 DROPS LAVENDER

3 DROPS LEMON

3 DROPS ORANGE

NAME: CLEANLINESS

5 DROPS BERGAMOT

3 DROPS LEMON

3 DROPS SPEARMINT

NAME: BREATH OF AIR

3 DROPS LAVENDER

3 DROPS LEMON

3 DROPS PEPPERMINT

NAME: FRESH FLOWERS

4 DROPS GRAPFRUIT

3 DROPS GERANIUM

3 DROPS LAVENDER

NAME: GARDEN FRESH

4 DROPS ROSEMARY

2 DROPS YLANG-YLANG

2 DROPS LAVENDER

NAME: NATURAL WONDER

4 DROPS PALMAROSA

3 DROPS SPEARMINT

3 DROPS CLARY-SAGE

NAME: SEASIDE

2 DROPS LAVENDER

2 DROPS PEPPERMINT

2 DROPS ROSEMARY

NOTES:

Testing Out Blends

NAME: _____

PURPOSE:

INGREDIENTS:

DIFFUSER

INHALER

TOPICAL

OTHER

MY RATING:

NOTES:

Testing Out Blends

NAME: **PURPOSE**:

INGREDIENTS:

DIFFUSER

INHALER

TOPICAL

OTHER

MY RATING:

NOTES:

My Favorite Blends

NAME: USED FOR:

INGREDIENTS:

NOTES:

NAME: USED FOR:

INGREDIENTS:

NOTES:

Essential Oil Recipes

NAME:

NAME:

NAME:

NAME:

NAME:

NAME:

NAME:

NAME:

Day to Day Blends

DIFFUSER BLENDS

NAME: RENEWAL

4 DROPS EUCALYPTUS

2 DROPS FRANKINCENSE

1 DROPS VETIVER

NAME: SUNNY SKIES

4 DROPS GRAPEFRUIT

4 DROPS ORANGE

2 DROPS BERGAMOT

NAME: BREATHE FREELY

3 DROPS EUCALYPTUS

3 DROPS LEMON

3 DROPS PEPPERMINT

NAME: BATHROOM FRESH

4 DROPS EUCALYPTUS

3 DROPS PEPPERMINT

2 DROPS TEA TREE

NAME: COLD FIGHTER

4 DROPS LAVENDER

4 DROPS EUCALYPTUS

2 DROPS TEA TREE

NAME: SHOWER POWER

5 DROPS LEMON

4 DROPS GRAPEFRUIT

2 DROPS PEPPERMINT

NAME: BREATHE EASY

4 DROPS PEPPERMINT

2 DROPS EUCALYPTUS

2 DROPS LEMON

NAME: SQUEAKY CLEAN

4 DROPS EUCALYPTUS

4 DROPS LEMON

2 DROPS CYPRUS

NOTES:

My Favorite Oils

VALENTINE'S DAY

SPRING

SUMMER

AUTUMN

HALLOWEEN

WINTER

CHRISTMAS

NEW YEARS

My Oil Ratings

PURPOSE OF OIL

NAME:

MY RATING:

PURPOSE OF OIL

NAME:

MY RATING:

PURPOSE OF OIL

NAME:

MY RATING:

PURPOSE OF OIL

NAME:

MY RATING:

PURPOSE OF OIL

NAME:

MY RATING:

NOTES:

Testing Out Blends

NAME:

PURPOSE:

INGREDIENTS:

DIFFUSER

INHALER

TOPICAL

OTHER

MY RATING:

NOTES:

Testing Out Blends

NAME:

PURPOSE:

INGREDIENTS:

DIFFUSER

INHALER

TOPICAL

OTHER

MY RATING:

NOTES:

My Favorite Blends

NAME: USED FOR:

INGREDIENTS:

NOTES:

NAME: USED FOR:

INGREDIENTS:

NOTES:

Essential Oil Recipes

NAME:

NAME:

NAME:

NAME:

NAME:

NAME:

NAME:

NAME:

Blends That Work Best For Me

DIFFUSER BLENDS

NAME:

NAME:

NAME:

NAME:

NAME:

NAME:

NAME:

NAME:

NOTES:

Perfume Blend Suggestions

ROLL-ON BLENDS TO BE DILUTED WITH 1 OZ. CARRIER OIL

NAME: SWEET SENSATION

3 DROPS YLANG-YLANG

4 DROPS BERGAMOT

2 DROPS LIME

NAME: CITRUS BOUQUET

4 DROPS SWEET ORANGE

3 DROPS JASMINE

3 DROPS LIME

NAME: WANDERLUST

5 DROPS BERGAMOT

3 DROPS SANDALWOOD

3 DROPS VANILLA

NAME: THE WOODSMAN

4 DROPS JUNIPER

4 DROPS CYPRESS

4 DROPS PINE

NAME: STAR-CROSSED

4 DROPS YLANG-YLANG

4 DROPS JASMINE

3 DROPS ROSE

NAME: TWILIGHT KISSES

4 DROPS BERGAMOT

2 DROPS PATCHOULI

3 DROPS YLANG-YLANG

NAME: TRUE LOVE

6 DROPS VANILLA

3 DROPS SANDALWOOD

2 DROPS ROSE

NAME: UNFORGETTABLE

5 DROPS SANDALWOOD

3 DROPS CINNAMON

3 DROPS PATCHOULI

NOTES: EXAMPLES OF CARRIER OILS ARE ALMOND,, APRICOT KERNEL, GRAPESEED, ROSEHIP,, OR COCONUT OIL. TYPICAL DILUTION IS 1-2 DROPS ESSENTIAL OIL FOR 1 TSP CARRIER OIL. DILUTION INSTRUCTIONS ARE FOR THE AVERAGE PERSON AND NOT FOR PREGNANT WOMEN, CHILDREN, PETS, OR THE ELDERLY. **ALWAYS CONSULT A DOCTOR PRIOR TO USING ESSENTIAL OILS.** IF EXPERIENCING IRRITATION, DISCONTINUE USE.

Testing Out Blends

NAME:

PURPOSE:

INGREDIENTS:

DIFFUSER

INHALER

TOPICAL

OTHER

MY RATING:

NOTES:

Testing Out Blends

NAME:

PURPOSE:

INGREDIENTS:

DIFFUSER

INHALER

TOPICAL

OTHER

MY RATING:

NOTES:

My Favorite Perfume Blends

PERFUME BLENDS

NAME:

NAME:

NAME:

NAME:

NAME:

NAME:

NAME:

NAME:

NOTES:

My Favorite Magical Oils

THE GODS

THE GODDESSES

LUCK

MONEY

LOVE

INSPIRATION

DIVINATION

PROTECTION

My Favorite Magical Oils

GRATITUDE

COURAGE

Magical Blends

DIFFUSER BLENDS

NAME: SACRED CIRCLE

6 DROPS LEMON

4 DROPS CYPRESS

3 DROPS ROSEMARY

NAME: SEA WITCH

4 DROPS LIME

3 DROPS LAVENDER

3 DROPS SPEARMINT

NAME: SPELLBOUND

4 DROPS PATCHOULI

3 DROPS SANDALWOOD

2 DROPS LAVENDER

NAME: RABBIT'S FOOT

3 DROPS ROSEMARY

2 DROPS CEDARWOOD

2 DROPS LEMON

NAME: WITCH'S SONG

4 DROPS PATCHOULI

2 DROPS CINNAMON

2 DROPS CEDAR

NAME: MOON MAIDEN

5 DROPS CEDARWOOD

4 DROPS LIME

3 DROPS EUCALYPTUS

NAME: DIVINE KNOWLEDGE

2 DROPS FRANKINCENSE

2 DROPS ROSEMARY

2 DROPS PEPPERMINT

NAME: WARRIOR'S SHIELD

6 DROPS CLOVE

5 DROPS LEMON

3 DROPS CINNAMON

NOTES:

Testing Out Blends

NAME: **PURPOSE**:

INGREDIENTS:

| |
| |

DIFFUSER

INHALER

TOPICAL

OTHER

MY RATING:

NOTES:

My Favorite Magical Blends

NAME:

USED FOR:

INGREDIENTS:

NOTES:

NAME:

USED FOR:

INGREDIENTS:

NOTES:

My Best Essential Oil Recipes

NAME:

NAME:

NAME:

NAME:

NAME:

NAME:

NAME:

NAME:

Essential Oil Wish List

NAME	USED FOR	PRICE	KID SAFE?

Essential Oil Wish List

NAME	USED FOR	PRICE	KID SAFE?

www.ingramcontent.com/pod-product-compliance
Lightning Source LLC
Chambersburg PA
CBHW051350280526
45784CB00007B/2896